Air Fryer Cooking Guide for Beginners

Boost Your Metabolism and Enjoy Your Meals with Incredibly Tasty Air Fryer Dishes

Eva Sheppard

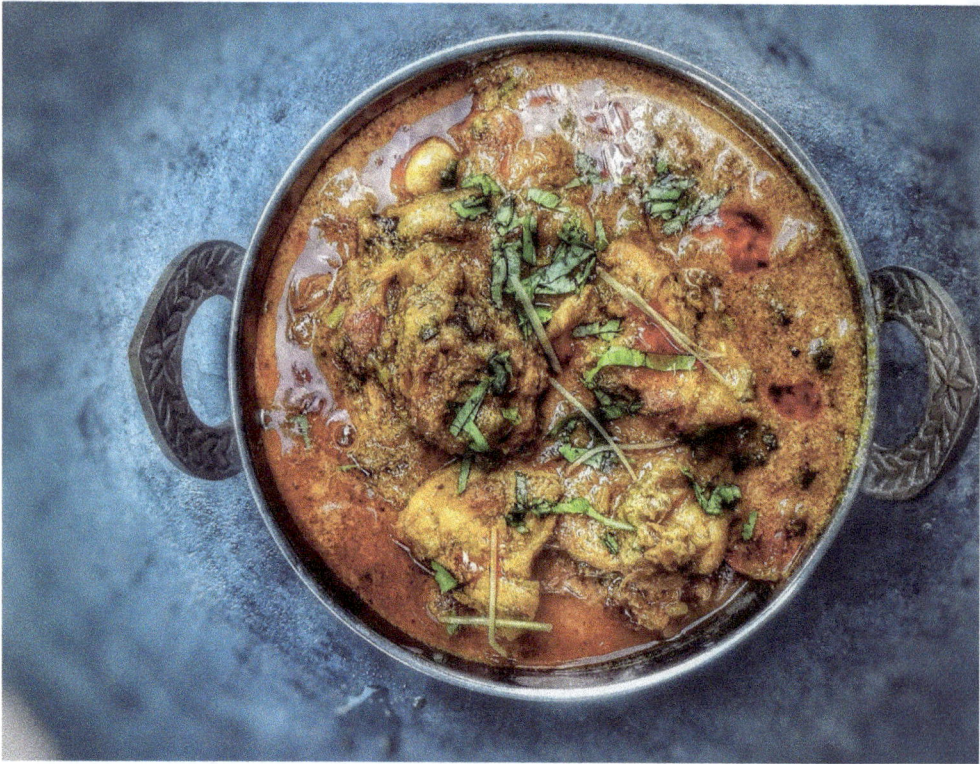

TABLE OF CONTENT

Pork Chops and Green Beans Recipe

Preparation Time: 25 Minutes

Servings: 4

Ingredients:

- 4 pork chops; bone in
- 2 tbsp. olive oil
- 16 oz. green beans
- 3 garlic cloves; minced
- 2 tbsp. parsley; chopped
- 1 tbsp. sage; chopped
- Salt and black pepper to the taste

Directions:

1. In a pan that fits your air fryer, mix pork chops with olive oil, sage, salt, pepper, green beans, garlic and parsley, toss, introduce in your air fryer and cook at 360 °F, for 15 minutes

2. Divide everything on plates and serve

Nutrition Values: Calories: 261; Fat: 7; Fiber: 9; Carbs: 14; Protein: 20

Asian Pork Recipe

Preparation Time: 45 Minutes

Servings: 4

Ingredients:

- 1 tsp. ginger powder
- 2 tsp. chili paste
- 2 garlic cloves; minced
- 2 tbsp. olive oil
- 3 oz. peanuts; ground
- 3 tbsp. soy sauce
- 1 shallot; chopped
- 1 tsp. coriander; ground
- 14 oz. pork chops; cubed
- 7 oz. coconut milk
- Salt and black pepper to the taste

Directions:

1. In a bowl; mix ginger with 1 tsp. chili paste, half of the garlic, half of the soy sauce and half of the oil, whisk, add meat, toss and leave aside for 10 minutes.

2. Transfer meat to your air fryer's basket and cook at 400 °F, for 12 minutes; turning halfway.

3. Meanwhile; heat up a pan with the rest of the oil over medium high heat, add shallot, the rest of the garlic, coriander, coconut milk, the rest of the peanuts, the rest of the chili paste and the rest of the soy sauce; stir and cook for 5 minutes. Divide pork on plates, spread coconut mix on top and serve.

Nutrition Values: Calories: 423; Fat: 11; Fiber: 4; Carbs: 42; Protein: 18

Spiced Pork Chops

Preparation time: 5 minutes

Cooking time: 15 minutes

Servings: 4

Ingredients:

- 4 medium pork chops
- Salt and black pepper to taste
- 1 tablespoon olive oil
- 2 tablespoons sweet paprika
- 2 tablespoons onion powder
- 2 tablespoons garlic powder
- 2 tablespoons oregano, dried
- 1 tablespoon cumin, ground
- 1 tablespoon rosemary, dried

Directions:

1. In a bowl, mix all of the ingredients and rub the pork chops well.

2. Put the pork chops in your air fryer's basket and cook at 400 degrees F for 15 minutes, flipping them halfway.

3. Divide between plates, serve, and enjoy.

Nutrition Values: calories 281, fat 8, fiber 7, carbs 17, protein 19

Chinese Pork and Broccoli Mix

Preparation time: 5 minutes

Cooking time: 15 minutes

Servings: 4

Ingredients:

- 1 pound pork stew meat, cut into strips
- 1 pound broccoli florets
- ⅓ cup oyster sauce
- 2 teaspoons olive oil
- 1 teaspoon soy sauce
- 1 garlic clove, minced

Directions:

1. In a bowl, mix the pork with all the other ingredients and toss well.

2. Put the mixture into your air fryer and cook at 390 degrees F for 15 minutes.

3. Divide into bowls and serve.

Nutrition Values: calories 281, fat 12, fiber 7, carbs 19, protein 20

French Beef Mix

Preparation time: 5 minutes

Cooking time: 15 minutes

Servings: 2

Ingredients:

- 1 red onion, sliced
- 1 green bell pepper, cut in strips
- Salt and black pepper to taste
- 2 teaspoons Provencal herbs
- ½ tablespoon mustard
- 1 tablespoon olive oil
- 7 ounces beef fillets, cut into strips

Directions:

1. Place all the ingredients in a baking dish that fits your air fryer and mix well.

2. Put the pan in the fryer and cook at 400 degrees F for 15 minutes.

3. Divide the mixture between bowls and serve.

Nutrition Values: calories 291, fat 8, fiber 7, carbs 19, protein 20

Beef and Mushroom Mix

Preparation time: 5 minutes

Cooking time: 17 minutes

Servings: 2

Ingredients:

- 2 beef steaks, cut into strips
- Salt and black pepper to taste
- 8 ounces white mushrooms, sliced
- 1 yellow onion, chopped
- 2 tablespoons dark soy sauce
- 1 teaspoon olive oil

Directions:

1. In a baking dish that fits your air fryer, combine all ingredients; toss well.

2. Place the pan in the fryer and cook at 390 degrees F for 17 minutes.

3. Divide everything between plates and serve.

Nutrition Values: calories 285, fat 8, fiber 2, carbs 18, protein 20

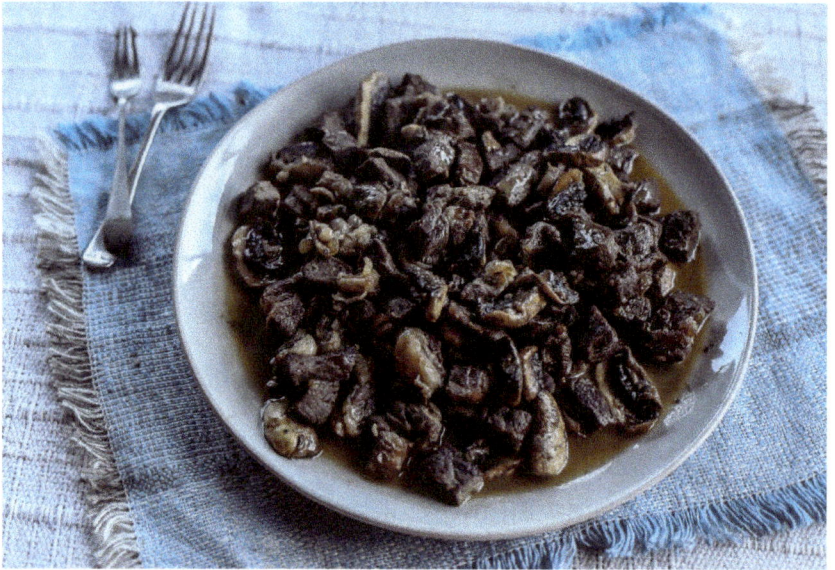

Oregano Pork Chops

Preparation time: 5 minutes

Cooking time: 15 minutes

Servings: 4

Ingredients:

- 2 tablespoons olive oil

- 4 pork chops

- Salt and black pepper to taste

- 4 garlic cloves, minced

- 2 tablespoon oregano, chopped

Directions:

1. Place all of the ingredients in a bowl and toss / mix well.

2. Transfer the chops to your air fryer's basket and cook at 400 degrees F for 15 minutes.

3. Serve with a side salad and enjoy!

Nutrition Values: calories 301, fat 7, fiber 5, carbs 19, protein 22

Crusted Rack of Lamb

Preparation time: 10 minutes

Cooking time: 20 minutes

Servings: 4

Ingredients:

- 2 tablespoons macadamia nuts, toasted and crushed
- 1 tablespoon vegetable oil
- 2 garlic cloves, minced
- 28 ounces rack of lamb
- Salt and black pepper to taste
- 1 egg, whisked
- 1 tablespoon oregano, chopped

Directions:

1. In a bowl, mix the lamb with the salt, pepper, garlic, and the oil; rub the lamb well.

2. In another bowl, mix the macadamia nuts with the oregano, salt, and pepper; stir.

3. Put the egg in a third bowl.

4. Dredge the lamb in the egg, then in the macadamia nuts mix.

5. Place the lamb in your air fryer's basket and cook at 380 degrees F for 10 minutes on each side.

6. Divide between plates and serve with a side salad.

Nutrition Values: calories 280, fat 12, fiber 8, carbs 20, protein 19

Coconut Pork Mix

Preparation time: 5 minutes

Cooking time: 15 minutes

Servings: 4

Ingredients:

- 1 teaspoon ginger, grated
- 2 teaspoons chili paste
- 2 garlic cloves, minced
- 14 ounces pork chops, cut into strips
- 1 shallot, chopped
- 7 ounces coconut milk
- 2 tablespoons olive oil
- 3 tablespoons soy sauce
- Salt and black pepper to taste

Directions:

1. In a baking dish that fits your air fryer, mix the pork with the ginger, chili paste, garlic, shallots, oil soy sauce, salt, and pepper; toss well.

2. Place the pan in the fryer and cook at 400 degrees F for 12 minutes, shaking the fryer halfway.

3. Add the coconut milk, toss, and cook for 3-4 minutes more.

4. Divide everything into bowls and serve.

Nutrition Values: calories 283, fat 11, fiber 9, carbs 22, protein 14

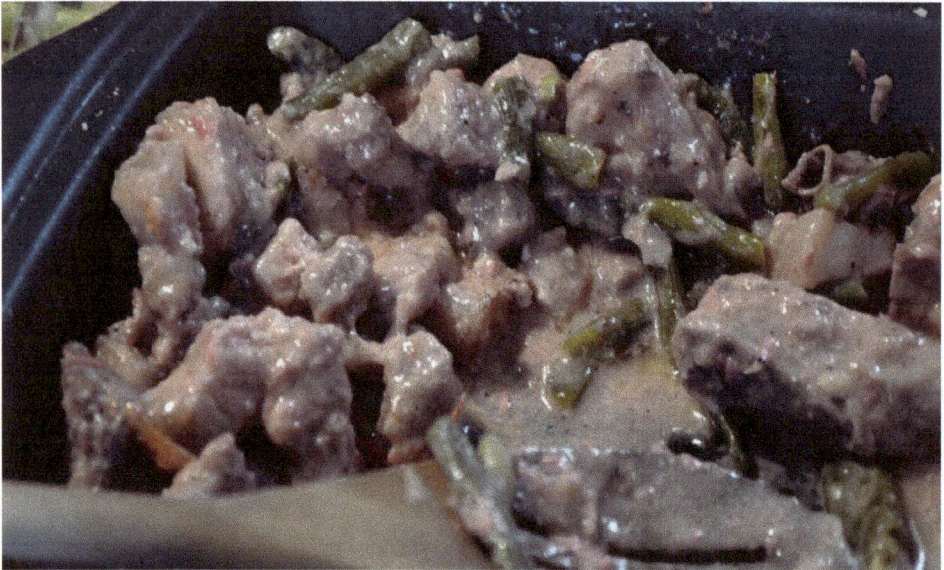

Creamy Pork and Sprouts

Preparation time: 10 minutes

Cooking time: 25 minutes

Servings: 4

Ingredients:

- 1 pound pork tenderloin, cubed
- 2 tablespoons olive oil
- 2 tablespoons rosemary, chopped
- Salt and black pepper to taste
- 1 garlic clove, minced
- 1½ pounds Brussels sprouts, trimmed
- ½ cup sour cream
- Salt and black pepper to taste

Directions:

1. In a pan that fits your air fryer, mix the pork with the oil, rosemary, salt, pepper, garlic, salt, and pepper; toss well.

2. Place the pan in the fryer and cook at 400 degrees F for 17 minutes.

3. Next add the sprouts and the sour cream and toss.

4. Place the pan in the fryer and cook for 8 more minutes.

5. Divide everything into bowls and serve.

Nutrition Values: calories 280, fat 13, fiber 9, carbs 22, protein 18

Pork and Chives Mix

Preparation time: 10 minutes

Cooking time: 22 minutes

Servings: 6

Ingredients:

- 1 cup mayonnaise
- 2 garlic cloves, minced
- 1 pound pork tenderloin, cubed
- 2 tablespoons chives, chopped
- 2 tablespoons mustard
- ¼ cup tarragon, chopped
- Salt and black pepper to taste

Directions:

1. Place all ingredients except the mayo into a pan that fits your air fryer; mix well.

2. Put the pan in the fryer and cook at 400 degrees F for 15 minutes.

3. Add the mayo and toss.

4. Put the pan in the fryer for 7 more minutes.

5. Divide into bowls and serve.

Nutrition Values: calories 280, fat 12, fiber 2, carbs 17, protein 14

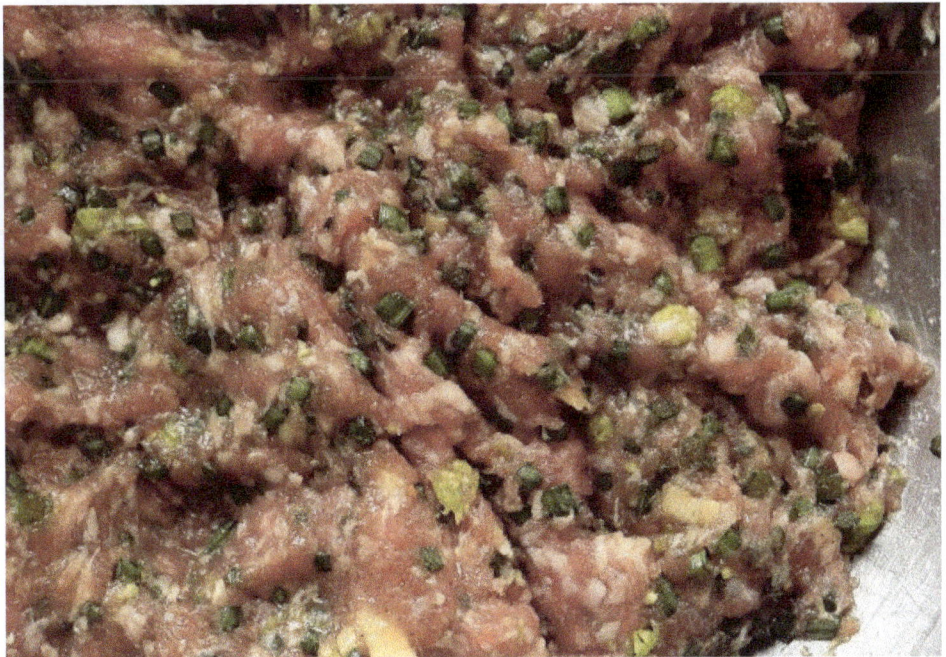

Beef and Wine Sauce

Preparation time: 10 minutes

Cooking time: 40 minutes

Servings: 6

Ingredients:

- 2 tablespoons butter, melted
- 3 garlic cloves, minced
- Salt and black pepper to taste
- 1 tablespoon mustard
- 3 pounds beef roast
- 1¾ cups beef stock
- ¾ cup red wine

Directions:

1. In a bowl, mix the beef with the butter, mustard, garlic, salt, and pepper; rub the meat thoroughly.

2. Put the beef roast in your air fryer's basket and cook at 400 degrees F for 15 minutes.

3. Heat up a pan over medium-high heat and add the stock and the wine.

4. Then add the beef roast and place the pan in the fryer; cook at 380 degrees F for 25 minutes more.

5. Divide into bowls and serve.

Nutrition Values: calories 300, fat 11, fiber 4, carbs 18, protein 22

Lamb Chops and Dill

Preparation time: 10 minutes

Cooking time: 20 minutes

Servings: 6

Ingredients:

- 1 pound lamb chops
- 2 yellow onions, chopped
- 1 tablespoon olive oil
- 1 garlic clove, minced
- 3 cups chicken stock
- 2 tablespoons sweet paprika
- Salt and black pepper to taste
- 1½ cups heavy cream
- 2 tablespoons dill, chopped

Directions:

1. Put the lamb chops in your air fryer and season with the salt, pepper, garlic, and paprika; rub the chops thoroughly.

2. Cook at 380 degrees F for 10 minutes.

3. Transfer the lamb to a baking dish that fits your air fryer. Then add the onions, stock, cream, and dill, and toss.

4. Place the pan in the fryer and cook everything for 7-8 minutes more.

5. Divide everything between plates and serve hot.

Nutrition Values: calories 310, fat 8, fiber 10, carbs 19, protein 25

Mustard Pork Chops

Preparation time: 10 minutes

Cooking time: 15 minutes

Servings: 6

Ingredients:

- 2 pork chops
- ¼ cup olive oil
- 2 garlic cloves, minced
- 1 tablespoon mustard
- 1 teaspoon sweet paprika
- Salt and black pepper to taste

Directions:

1. Place all of the ingredients in a bowl, and coat the pork chops well.

2. Transfer the pork chops to your air fryer's basket and cook at 400 degrees F for 15 minutes.

3. Divide the chops between plates and serve

Nutrition Values: calories 284, fat 14, fiber 4, carbs 17, protein 28

Flavored Rib Eye Steak

Preparation time: 10 minutes

Cooking time: 20 minutes

Servings: 4

Ingredients:

- 2 pounds rib eye steak
- Salt and black pepper to the taste
- 1 tablespoons olive oil

For the rub:

- 3 tablespoons sweet paprika
- 2 tablespoons onion powder
- 2 tablespoons garlic powder
- 1 tablespoon brown sugar
- 2 tablespoons oregano, dried
- 1 tablespoon cumin, ground
- 1 tablespoon rosemary, dried

Directions:

1. In a bowl, mix paprika with onion and garlic powder, sugar, oregano, rosemary, salt,

pepper and cumin, stir and rub steak with this mix.

2. Season steak with salt and pepper, rub again with the oil, put in your air fryer and cook at 400 degrees F for 20 minutes, flipping them halfway.

3. Transfer steak to a cutting board, slice and serve with a side salad.

4. Enjoy!

Nutrition Values: calories 320, fat 8, fiber 7, carbs 22, protein 21

Chinese Steak and Broccoli

Preparation time: 45 minutes

Cooking time: 12 minutes

Servings: 4

Ingredients:

- ¾ pound round steak, cut into strips
- 1 pound broccoli florets
- 1/3 cup oyster sauce
- 2 teaspoons sesame oil
- 1 teaspoon soy sauce
- 1 teaspoon sugar
- 1/3 cup sherry
- 1 tablespoon olive oil
- 1 garlic clove, minced

Directions:

1. In a bowl, mix sesame oil with oyster sauce, soy sauce, sherry and sugar, stir well, add beef, toss and leave aside for 30 minutes.

2. Transfer beef to a pan that fits your air fryer, also add broccoli, garlic and oil, toss

everything and cook at 380 degrees F for 12 minutes.

3. Divide among plates and serve.

4. Enjoy!

Nutrition Values: calories 330, fat 12, fiber 7, carbs 23, protein 23

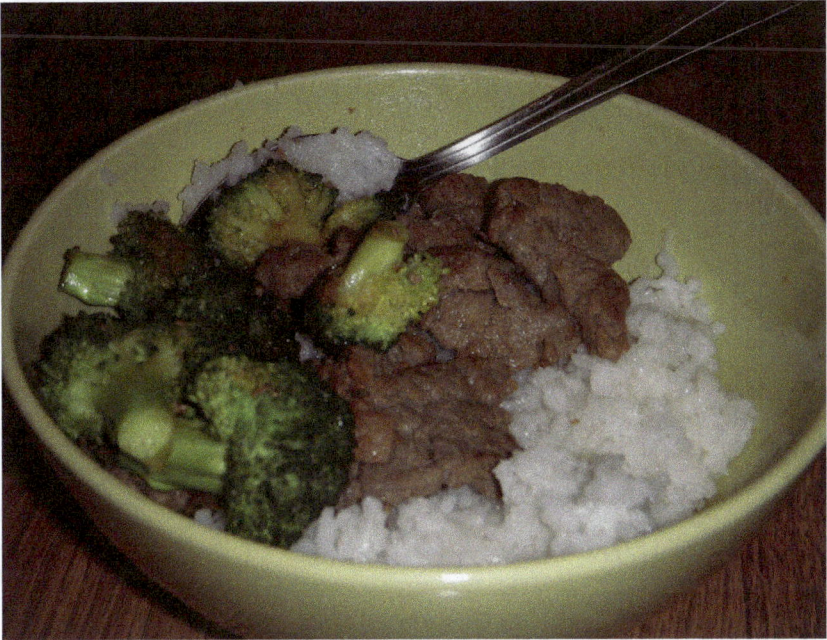

Provencal Pork

Preparation time: 10 minutes

Cooking time: 15 minutes

Servings: 2

Ingredients:

- 1 red onion, sliced
- 1 yellow bell pepper, cut into strips
- 1 green bell pepper, cut into strips
- Salt and black pepper to the taste
- 2 teaspoons Provencal herbs
- ½ tablespoon mustard
- 1 tablespoon olive oil
- 7 ounces pork tenderloin

Directions:

1. In a baking dish that fits your air fryer, mix yellow bell pepper with green bell pepper, onion, salt, pepper, Provencal herbs and half of the oil and toss well.

2. Season pork with salt, pepper, mustard and the rest of the oil, toss well and add to veggies.

3. Introduce everything in your air fryer, cook at 370 degrees F for 15 minutes, divide among plates and serve.

4. Enjoy!

Nutrition Values: calories 300, fat 8, fiber 7, carbs 21, protein 23

Beef Strips with Snow Peas and Mushrooms

Preparation time: 10 minutes

Cooking time: 22 minutes

Servings: 2

Ingredients:

- 2 beef steaks, cut into strips
- Salt and black pepper to the taste
- 7 ounces snow peas
- 8 ounces white mushrooms, halved
- 1 yellow onion, cut into rings
- 2 tablespoons soy sauce
- 1 teaspoon olive oil

Directions:

1. In a bowl, mix olive oil with soy sauce, whisk, add beef strips and toss.

2. In another bowl, mix snow peas, onion and mushrooms with salt, pepper and the oil, toss well, put in a pan that fits your air fryer and cook at 350 degrees F for 16 minutes.

3. Add beef strips to the pan as well and cook at 400 degrees F for 6 minutes more.

4. Divide everything on plates and serve.

5. Enjoy!

Nutrition Values: calories 235, fat 8, fiber 2, carbs 22, protein 24

Garlic Lamb Chops

Preparation time: 10 minutes

Cooking time: 10 minutes

Servings: 4

Ingredients:

- 3 tablespoons olive oil
- 8 lamb chops
- Salt and black pepper to the taste
- 4 garlic cloves, minced
- 1 tablespoon oregano, chopped
- 1 tablespoon coriander, chopped

Directions:

1. In a bowl, mix oregano with salt, pepper, oil, garlic and lamb chops and toss to coat.

2. Transfer lamb chops to your air fryer and cook at 400 degrees F for 10 minutes.

3. Divide lamb chops on plates and serve with a side salad.

4. Enjoy!

Nutrition Values: calories 231, fat 7, fiber 5, carbs 14, protein 23

Crispy Lamb

Preparation time: 10 minutes

Cooking time: 30 minutes

Servings: 4

Ingredients:

- 1 tablespoon bread crumbs
- 2 tablespoons macadamia nuts, toasted and crushed
- 1 tablespoon olive oil
- 1 garlic clove, minced
- 28 ounces rack of lamb
- Salt and black pepper to the taste
- 1 egg,
- 1 tablespoon rosemary, chopped

Directions:

1. In a bowl, mix oil with garlic and stir well.

2. Season lamb with salt, pepper and brush with the oil.

3. In another bowl, mix nuts with breadcrumbs and rosemary.

4. Put the egg in a separate bowl and whisk well.

5. Dip lamb in egg, then in macadamia mix, place them in your air fryer's basket, cook at 360 degrees F and cook for 25 minutes, increase heat to 400 degrees F and cook for 5 minutes more.

6. Divide among plates and serve right away.

7. Enjoy!

Nutrition Values: calories 230, fat 2, fiber 2, carbs 10, protein 12

Indian Pork

Preparation time: 35 minutes

Cooking time: 10 minutes

Servings: 4

Ingredients:

- 1 teaspoon ginger powder
- 2 teaspoons chili paste
- 2 garlic cloves, minced
- 14 ounces pork chops, cubed
- 1 shallot, chopped
- 1 teaspoon coriander, ground
- 7 ounces coconut milk
- 2 tablespoons olive oil
- 3 ounces peanuts, ground
- 3 tablespoons soy sauce
- Salt and black pepper to the taste

Directions:

1. In a bowl, mix ginger with 1 teaspoon chili paste, half of the garlic, half of the soy sauce and half of the oil, whisk, add meat, toss and leave aside for 10 minutes.

2. Transfer meat to your air fryer's basket and cook at 400 degrees F for 12 minutes, turning halfway.

3. Meanwhile, heat up a pan with the rest of the oil over medium high heat, add shallot, the rest of the garlic, coriander, coconut milk, the rest of the peanuts, the rest of the chili paste and the rest of the soy sauce, stir and cook for 5 minutes.

4. Divide pork on plates, spread coconut mix on top and serve.

5. Enjoy!

Nutrition Values: calories 423, fat 11, fiber 4, carbs 42, protein 18

Lamb and Creamy Brussels Sprouts

Preparation time: 10 minutes

Cooking time: 1 hour and 10 minutes

Servings: 4

Ingredients:

- 2 pounds leg of lamb, scored
- 2 tablespoons olive oil
- 1 tablespoon rosemary, chopped
- 1 tablespoon lemon thyme, chopped
- 1 garlic clove, minced
- 1 and ½ pounds Brussels sprouts, trimmed
- 1 tablespoon butter, melted
- ½ cup sour cream
- Salt and black pepper to the taste

Directions:

1. Season leg of lamb with salt, pepper, thyme and rosemary, brush with oil, place in your air fryer's basket, cook at 300 degrees F for 1 hour, transfer to a plate and keep warm.

2. In a pan that fits your air fryer, mix Brussels sprouts with salt, pepper, garlic, butter and sour cream, toss, put in your air fryer and cook at 400 degrees F for 10 minutes.

3. Divide lamb on plates, add Brussels sprouts on the side and serve.

4. Enjoy!

Nutrition Values: calories 440, fat 23, fiber 0, carbs 2, protein 49

Beef Fillets with Garlic Mayo

Preparation time: 10 minutes

Cooking time: 40 minutes

Servings: 8

Ingredients:

- 1 cup mayonnaise
- 1/3 cup sour cream
- 2 garlic cloves, minced
- 3 pounds beef fillet
- 2 tablespoons chives, chopped
- 2 tablespoons mustard
- 2 tablespoons mustard
- ¼ cup tarragon, chopped
- Salt and black pepper to the taste

Directions:

1. Season beef with salt and pepper to the taste, place in your air fryer, cook at 370 degrees F for 20 minutes, transfer to a plate and leave aside for a few minutes.

2. In a bowl, mix garlic with sour cream, chives, mayo, some salt and pepper, whisk and leave aside.

3. In another bowl, mix mustard with Dijon mustard and tarragon, whisk, add beef, toss, return to your air fryer and cook at 350 degrees F for 20 minutes more.

4. Divide beef on plates, spread garlic mayo on top and serve.

5. Enjoy!

Nutrition Values: calories 400, fat 12, fiber 2, carbs 27, protein 19

Mustard Marinated Beef

Preparation time: 10 minutes

Cooking time: 45 minutes

Servings: 6

Ingredients:

- 6 bacon strips
- 2 tablespoons butter
- 3 garlic cloves, minced
- Salt and black pepper to the taste
- 1 tablespoon horseradish
- 1 tablespoon mustard
- 3 pounds beef roast
- 1 and ¾ cup beef stock
- ¾ cup red wine

Directions:

1. In a bowl, mix butter with mustard, garlic, salt, pepper and horseradish, whisk and rub beef with this mix.

2. Arrange bacon strips on a cutting board, place beef on top, fold bacon around beef, transfer to your air fryer's basket, cook at

400 degrees F for 15 minutes and transfer to a pan that fits your fryer.

3. Add stock and wine to beef, introduce pan in your air fryer and cook at 360 degrees F for 30 minutes more.

4. Carve beef, divide among plates and serve with a side salad.

5. Enjoy!

Nutrition Values: calories 500, fat 9, fiber 4, carbs 29, protein 36

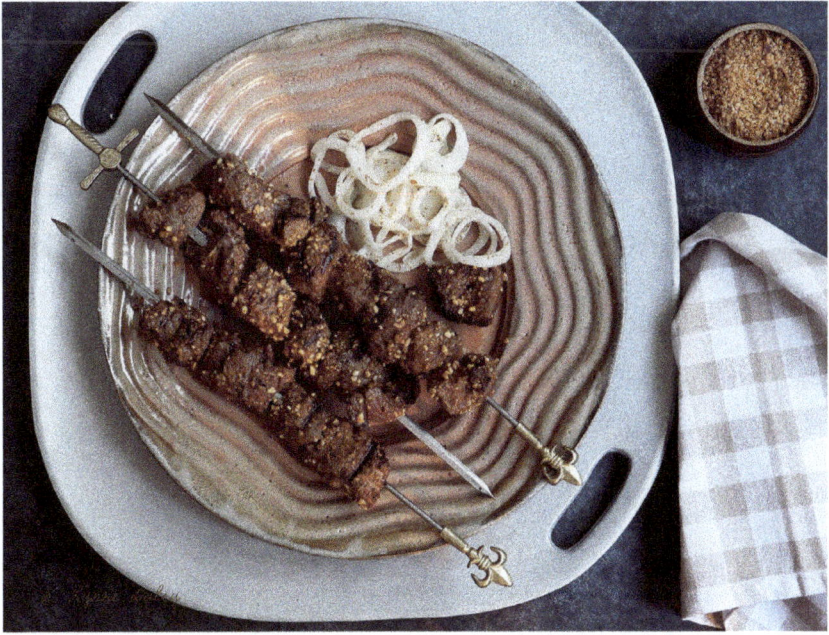

Creamy Pork

Preparation time: 10 minutes

Cooking time: 22 minutes

Servings: 6

Ingredients:

- 2 pounds pork meat, boneless and cubed
- 2 yellow onions, chopped
- 1 tablespoon olive oil
- 1 garlic clove, minced
- 3 cups chicken stock
- 2 tablespoons sweet paprika
- Salt and black pepper to the taste
- 2 tablespoons white flour
- 1 and ½ cups sour cream
- 2 tablespoons dill, chopped

Directions:

1. In a pan that fits your air fryer, mix pork with salt, pepper and oil, toss, introduce in your air fryer and cook at 360 degrees F for 7 minutes.

2. Add onion, garlic, stock, paprika, flour, sour cream and dill, toss and cook at 370 degrees F for 15 minutes more.

3. Divide everything on plates and serve right away.

4. Enjoy!

Nutrition Values: calories 300, fat 4, fiber 10, carbs 26, protein 34

Spinach and Cream Cheese Mix

Preparation time: 5 minutes

Cooking time: 8 minutes

Servings: 4

Ingredients:

- 14 ounces baby spinach
- 1 tablespoon olive oil
- 2 tablespoons milk
- 3 ounces cream cheese, softened
- Salt and black pepper to taste
- 1 yellow onion, chopped

Directions:

1. In a pan that fits your air fryer, mix all ingredients and toss gently.

2. Place the pan in the air fryer and cook at 260 degrees F for 8 minutes.

3. Divide between plates and serve.

Nutrition Values: calories 190, fat 4, fiber 2, carbs 13, protein 9

Chicken Curry

Preparation Time: 40 minutes

Servings: 4

Ingredients:

- 15 oz. chicken breast; skinless, boneless, cubed
- 6 potatoes; peeled and cubed
- 5 oz. heavy cream
- 1/2 bunch coriander; chopped
- 1 yellow onion; sliced
- 1 tbsp. olive oil
- 1 tsp. curry powder
- Salt and black pepper to taste

Directions:

1. Heat up the oil in a pan that fits your air fryer over medium heat.

2. Add the chicken, toss and brown for 2 minutes

3. Then add the onions, curry powder, salt and pepper; toss and cook for 3 minutes.

4. Next add the potatoes and the cream; toss well

5. Place the pan in the air fryer and cook at 370°F for 20 minutes

6. Add the coriander and stir. Divide the curry into bowls and serve.

Asian Atyle Chicken

Preparation Time: 40 minutes

Servings: 4

Ingredients:

- 1 lb. spinach; chopped.
- 1½ lbs. chicken drumsticks
- 15 oz. canned tomatoes; crushed
- 1/4 cup lemon juice
- 1/2 cup chicken stock
- 1/2 cup heavy cream
- 1/2 cup cilantro; chopped.
- 4 garlic cloves; minced
- 1 yellow onion; chopped.
- 2 tbsp. butter; melted
- 1 tbsp. ginger; grated
- 1½ tsp. coriander; ground
- 1½ tsp. paprika
- 1 tsp. turmeric powder
- Salt and black pepper to taste

Directions:

1. Place the butter in a pan that fits your air fryer and heat over medium heat.

2. Add the onions and the garlic, stir and cook for 3 minutes

3. Add the ginger, paprika, coriander, turmeric, salt, pepper and the chicken; toss and cook for 4 minutes more.

4. Add the tomatoes and the stock and stir

5. Place the pan in the fryer and cook at 370°F for 15 minutes

6. Add the spinach, lemon juice, cilantro and the cream; stir and cook for 5-6 minutes more. Divide everything into bowls and serve.

Lemongrass Chicken

Preparation Time: 40 minutes

Servings: 4

Ingredients:

- 10 chicken drumsticks
- 1 cup coconut milk
- 1 bunch lemongrass; trimmed
- 1/4 cup parsley; chopped.
- 1 yellow onion; chopped.
- 2 tbsp. fish sauce
- 3 tbsp. soy sauce
- 1 tsp. butter; melted
- 1 tbsp. ginger; chopped.
- 4 garlic cloves; minced
- 1 tbsp. lemon juice
- Salt and black pepper to taste

Directions:

1. In a blender, combine the lemongrass, ginger, garlic, soy sauce, fish sauce and coconut milk; pulse well.

2. Put the butter in a pan that fits your air fryer and heat it up over medium heat; add the onions, stir and cook for 2-3 minutes

3. Add the chicken, salt, pepper and the lemongrass mix; toss well

4. Place the pan in the fryer and cook at 380°F for 25 minutes

5. Add the lemon juice and the parsley and toss. Divide everything between plates and serve.

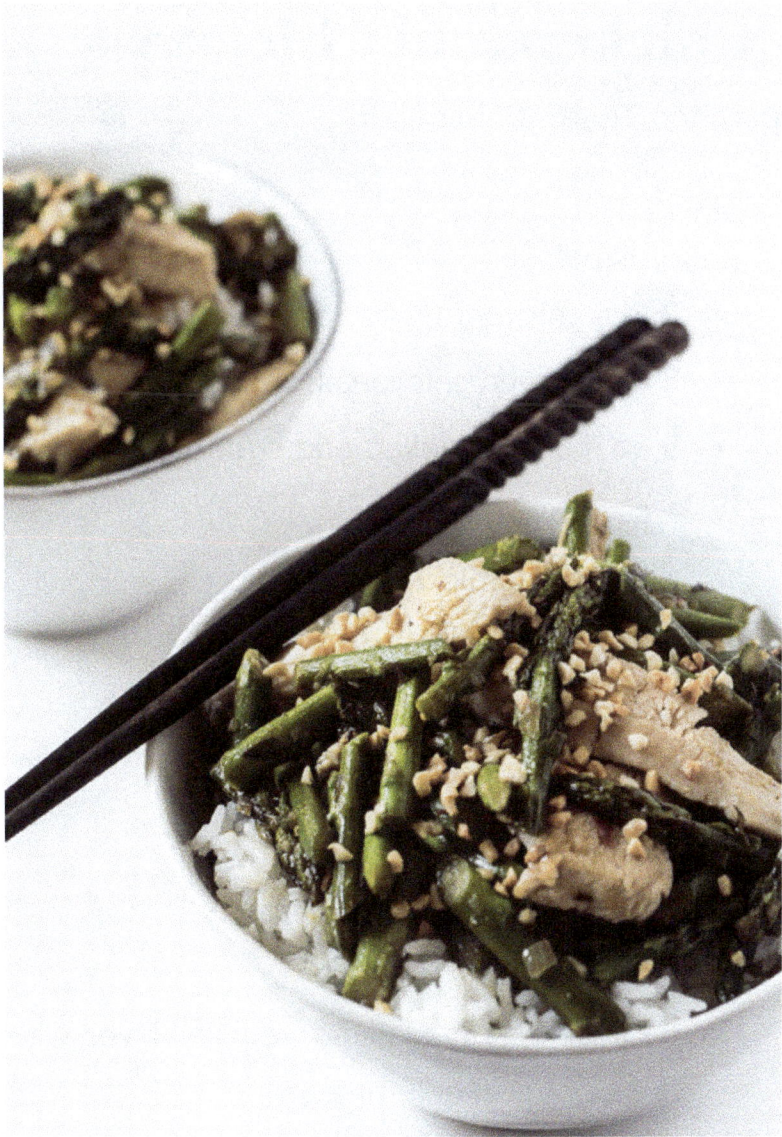

Chicken and Chickpeas

Preparation Time: 35 minutes

Servings: 4

Ingredients:

- 2 lbs. chicken thighs; boneless
- 8 oz. canned chickpeas; drained
- 5 oz. bacon; cooked and crumbled
- 1 cup chicken stock
- 1 tsp. balsamic vinegar
- 2 tbsp. olive oil
- 1 cup yellow onion; chopped.
- 2 carrots; chopped.
- 1 tbsp. parsley; chopped.
- Salt and black pepper to taste

Directions:

1. Heat up a pan that fits your air fryer with the oil over medium heat.

2. Add the onions, carrots, salt and pepper; stir and sauté for 3-4 minutes.

3. Add the chicken, stock, vinegar and chickpeas; then toss

4. Place the pan in the fryer and cook at 380°F for 20 minutes

5. Add the bacon and the parsley and toss again. Divide everything between plates and serve.

Pork with Couscous Recipe

Preparation Time: 45 Minutes

Servings: 6

Ingredients:

- 2 ½ lbs. pork loin; boneless and trimmed
- 2 ¼ tsp. sage; dried
- 3/4 cup chicken stock
- 1/2 tbsp. sweet paprika
- 1/2 tbsp. garlic powder
- 1/4 tsp. marjoram; dried
- 1/4 tsp. rosemary; dried
- 1 tsp. basil; dried
- 2 tbsp. olive oil
- 2 cups couscous; cooked
- 1 tsp. oregano; dried
- Salt and black pepper to the taste

Directions:

1. In a bowl; mix oil with stock, paprika, garlic powder, sage, rosemary, thyme, marjoram, oregano, salt and pepper to the

taste, whisk well, add pork loin, toss well and leave aside for 1 hour.

2. Transfer everything to a pan that fits your air fryer and cook at 370 °F, for 35 minutes. Divide among plates and serve with couscous on the side.

Nutrition Values: Calories: 310; Fat: 4; Fiber: 6; Carbs: 37; Protein: 34

Creamy Pork Recipe

Preparation Time: 32 Minutes

Servings: 6

Ingredients:

- 2 lbs. pork meat; boneless and cubed
- 2 yellow onions; chopped.
- 2 tbsp. dill; chopped.
- 2 tbsp. sweet paprika
- 1 tbsp. olive oil
- 1 garlic clove; minced
- 3 cups chicken stock
- 2 tbsp. white flour
- 1 ½ cups sour cream
- Salt and black pepper to the taste

Directions:

1. In a pan that fits your air fryer, mix pork with salt, pepper and oil, toss, introduce in your air fryer and cook at 360 °F, for 7 minutes.

2. Add onion, garlic, stock, paprika, flour, sour cream and dill, toss and cook at 370 °F, for

15 minutes more. Divide everything on plates and serve right away.

Nutrition Values: Calories: 300; Fat: 4; Fiber: 10; Carbs: 26; Protein: 34

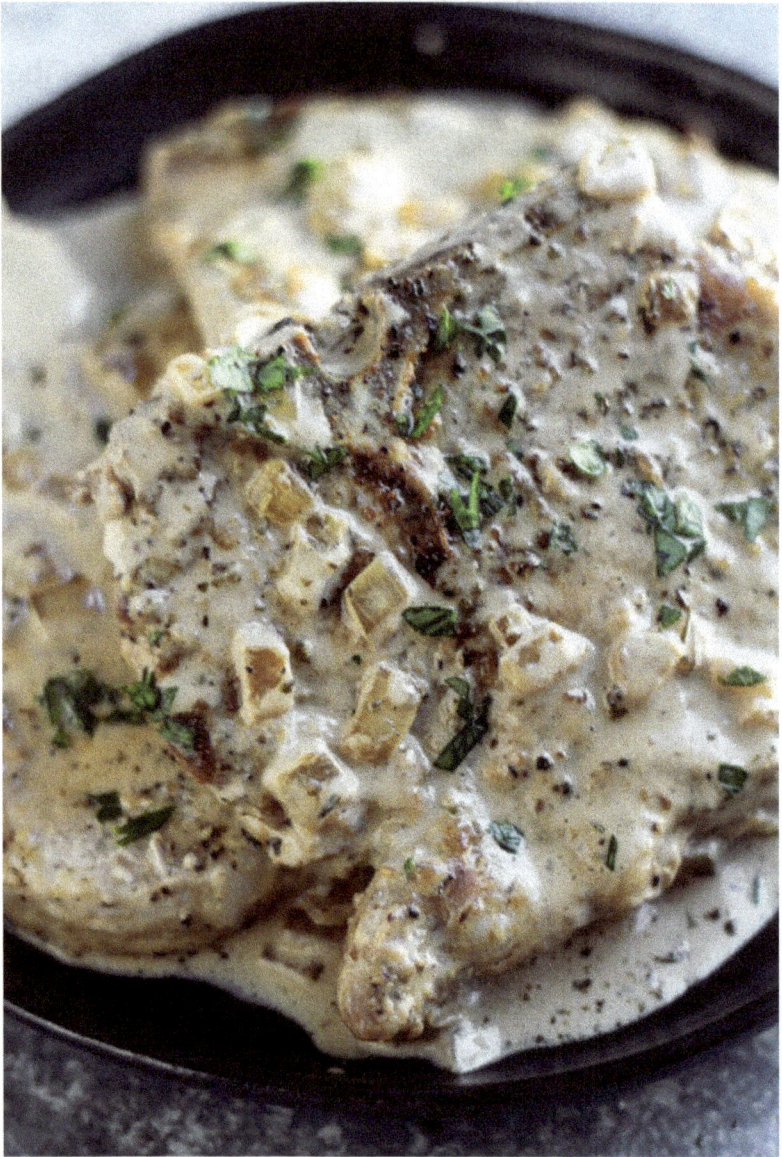

Lamb Roast and Potatoes Recipe

Preparation Time: 55 Minutes

Servings: 6

Ingredients:

- 4 lbs. lamb roast
- 4 bay leaves
- 3 garlic cloves; minced
- 1 spring rosemary
- 6 potatoes; halved
- 1/2 cup lamb stock
- Salt and black pepper to the taste

Directions:

1. Put potatoes in a dish that fits your air fryer, add lamb, garlic, rosemary spring, salt, pepper, bay leaves and stock, toss, introduce in your air fryer and cook at 360 °F, for 45 minutes. Slice lamb, divide among plates and serve with potatoes and cooking juices.

Nutrition Values: Calories: 273; Fat: 4; Fiber: 12; Carbs: 25; Protein: 29

Chinese Steak and Broccoli Recipe

Preparation Time: 57 Minutes

Servings: 4

Ingredients:

- 3/4 lb. round steak; cut into strips
- 1 lb. broccoli florets
- 1 tsp. sugar
- 1/3 cup sherry
- 1/3 cup oyster sauce
- 1 tbsp. olive oil
- 1 garlic clove; minced
- 2 tsp. sesame oil
- 1 tsp. soy sauce

Directions:

1. In a bowl; mix sesame oil with oyster sauce, soy sauce, sherry and sugar; stir well, add beef, toss and leave aside for 30 minutes.

2. Transfer beef to a pan that fits your air fryer, also add broccoli, garlic and oil, toss

everything and cook at 380 °F, for 12 minutes. Divide among plates and serve.

Nutrition Values: Calories: 330; Fat: 12; Fiber: 7; Carbs: 23; Protein: 23

Beef Fillets with Garlic Mayo Recipe

Preparation Time: 50 Minutes

Servings: 8

Ingredients:

- 3 lbs. beef fillet
- 1 cup mayonnaise
- 1/3 cup sour cream
- 2 tbsp. chives; chopped
- 2 tbsp. mustard
- 2 tbsp. mustard
- 1/4 cup tarragon; chopped
- 2 garlic cloves; minced
- Salt and black pepper to the taste

Directions:

1. Season beef with salt and pepper to the taste, place in your air fryer, cook at 370 °F, for 20 minutes; transfer to a plate and leave aside for a few minutes.

2. In a bowl; mix garlic with sour cream, chives, mayo, some salt and pepper, whisk and leave aside.

3. In another bowl, mix mustard with Dijon mustard and tarragon, whisk, add beef, toss, return to your air fryer and cook at 350 °F, for 20 minutes more. Divide beef on plates, spread garlic mayo on top and serve.

Nutrition Values: Calories: 400; Fat: 12; Fiber: 2; Carbs: 27; Protein: 19

Simple Braised Pork Recipe

Preparation Time: 1 hour 20 Minutes

Servings: 4

Ingredients:

- 2 lbs. pork loin roast; boneless and cubed
- 4 tbsp. butter; melted
- 2 cups chicken stock
- 1/2 lb. red grapes
- 1 bay leaf
- 1/2 yellow onion; chopped.
- 1/2 cup dry white wine
- 2 garlic cloves; minced
- 1 tsp. thyme; chopped
- 1 thyme spring
- 2 tbsp. white flour
- Salt and black pepper to the taste

Directions:

1. Season pork cubes with salt and pepper, rub with 2 tbsp. melted butter, put in your air fryer and cook at 370 °F, for 8 minutes.

2. Meanwhile; heat up a pan that fits your air fryer with 2 tbsp. butter over medium high heat, add garlic and onion; stir and cook for 2 minutes.

3. Add wine, stock, salt, pepper, thyme, flour and bay leaf; stir well, bring to a simmer and take off heat.

4. Add pork cubes and grapes, toss, introduce in your air fryer and cook at 360 °F, for 30 minutes more.

5. Divide everything on plates and serve.

Nutrition Values: Calories: 320; Fat: 4; Fiber: 5; Carbs: 29; Protein: 38

Lamb and Lemon Sauce Recipe

Preparation Time: 40 Minutes

Servings: 4

Ingredients:

- 2 lamb shanks
- 2 garlic cloves; minced
- 4 tbsp. olive oil
- Juice from 1/2 lemon
- Zest from 1/2 lemon
- 1/2 tsp. oregano; dried
- Salt and black pepper to the taste

Directions:

1. Season lamb with salt, pepper, rub with garlic, put in your air fryer and cook at 350 °F, for 30 minutes.

2. Meanwhile; in a bowl, mix lemon juice with lemon zest, some salt and pepper, the olive oil and oregano and whisk very well. Shred lamb, discard bone, divide among plates,

drizzle the lemon dressing all over and serve.

Nutrition Values: Calories: 260; Fat: 7; Fiber: 3; Carbs: 15; Protein: 12

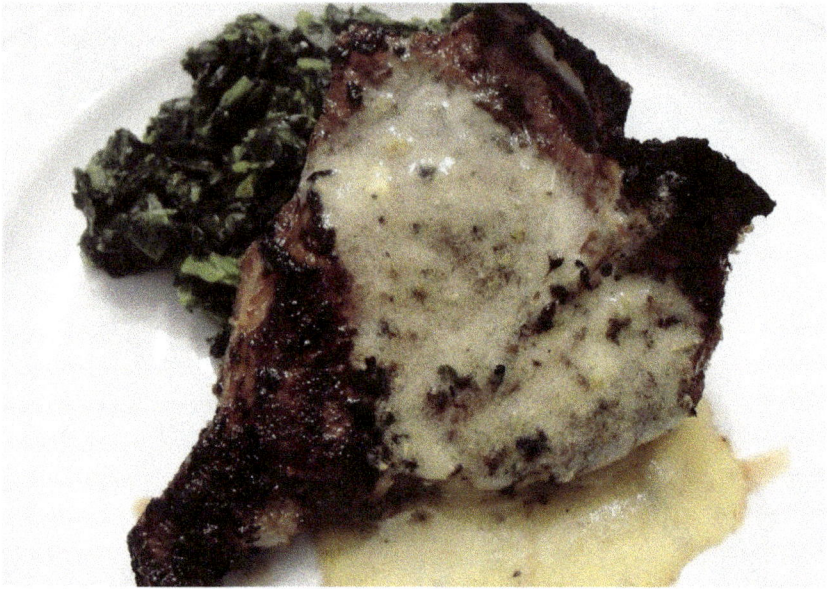

Provencal Pork Recipe

Preparation Time: 25 Minutes

Servings: 2

Ingredients:

- 7 oz. pork tenderloin
- 1 red onion; sliced
- 1 yellow bell pepper; cut into strips
- 2 tsp. Provencal herbs
- 1/2 tbsp. mustard
- 1 tbsp. olive oil
- 1 green bell pepper; cut into strips
- Salt and black pepper to the taste

Directions:

1. In a baking dish that fits your air fryer, mix yellow bell pepper with green bell pepper, onion, salt, pepper, Provencal herbs and half of the oil and toss well.

2. Season pork with salt, pepper, mustard and the rest of the oil, toss well and add to veggies. Introduce everything in your air fryer,

3. Cook at 370 °F, for 15 minutes; divide among plates and serve.

Nutrition Values: Calories: 300; Fat: 8; Fiber: 7; Carbs: 21; Protein: 23

Lemony Lamb Leg Recipe

Preparation Time: 1 hour 10 Minutes

Servings: 6

Ingredients:

- 4 lbs. lamb leg
- 2 tbsp. olive oil
- 2 springs rosemary; chopped.
- 2 tbsp. lemon juice
- 2 lbs. baby potatoes
- 1 cup beef stock
- 2 tbsp. parsley; chopped
- 2 tbsp. oregano; chopped
- 1 tbsp. lemon rind; grated
- 3 garlic cloves; minced
- Salt and black pepper to the taste

Directions:

1. Make small cuts all over lamb, insert rosemary springs and season with salt and pepper.

2. In a bowl; mix 1 tbsp. oil with oregano, parsley, garlic, lemon juice and rind; stir and rub lamb with this mix.

3. Heat up a pan that fits your air fryer with the rest of the oil over medium high heat, add potatoes; stir and cook for 3 minutes.

4. Add lamb and stock; stir, introduce in your air fryer and cook at 360 °F, for 1 hour. Divide everything on plates and serve.

Nutrition Values: Calories: 264; Fat: 4; Fiber: 12; Carbs: 27; Protein: 32

Beef Roast and Wine Sauce Recipe

Preparation Time: 55 Minutes

Servings: 6

Ingredients:

- 3 lbs. beef roast
- 17 oz. beef stock
- 4 garlic cloves; minced
- 3 carrots; chopped
- 5 potatoes; chopped
- 3 oz. red wine
- 1/2 tsp. chicken salt
- Salt and black pepper to the taste
- 1/2 tsp. smoked paprika
- 1 yellow onion; chopped

Directions:

1. In a bowl; mix salt, pepper, chicken salt and paprika; stir, rub beef with this mix and put it in a big pan that fits your air fryer.

2. Add onion, garlic, stock, wine, potatoes and carrots, introduce in your air fryer and cook

at 360 °F, for 45 minutes. Divide everything on plates and serve.

Nutrition Values: Calories: 304; Fat: 20; Fiber: 7; Carbs: 20; Protein: 32

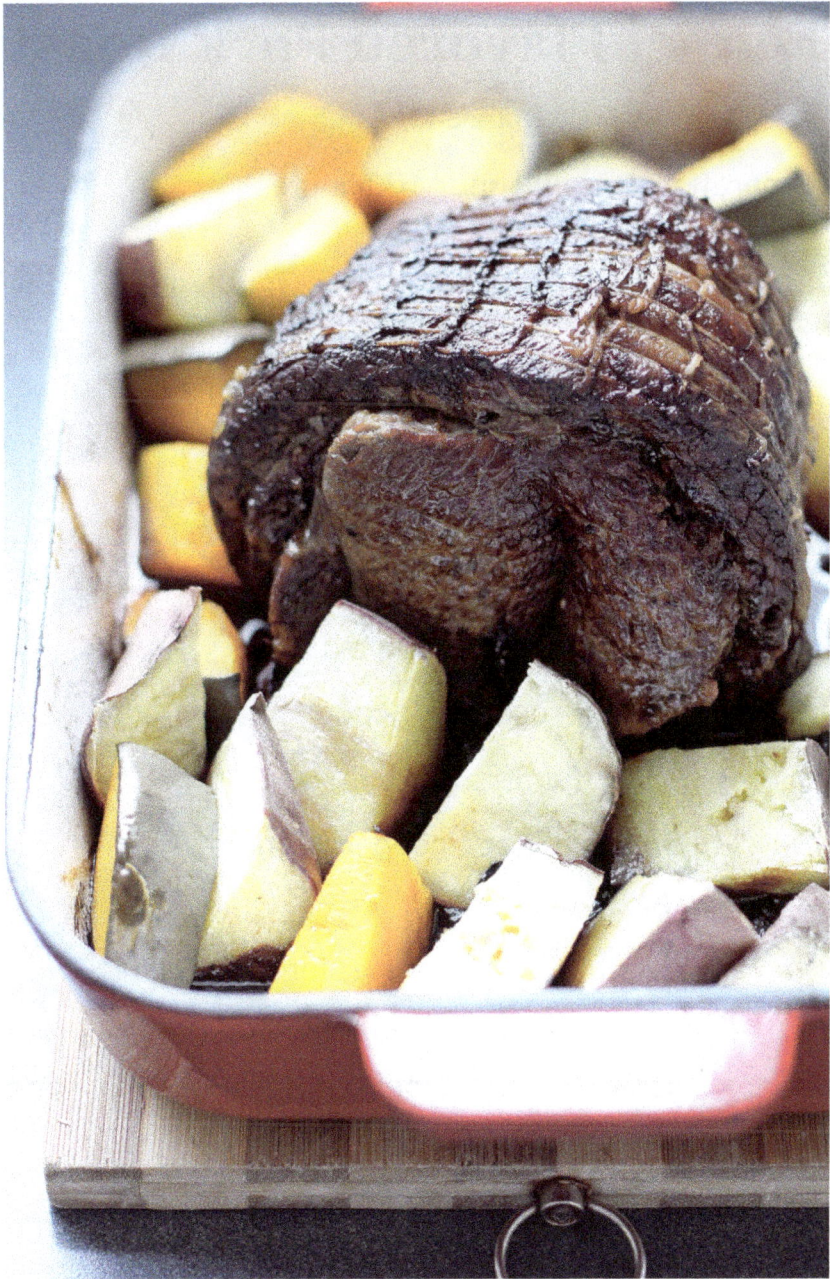

Fennel Flavored Pork Roast Recipe

Preparation Time: 1 hour 10 Minutes

Servings: 10

Ingredients:

- 5 ½ lbs. pork loin roast; trimmed
- 1 tbsp. fennel seeds
- 2 tsp. red pepper; crushed
- 1/4 cup olive oil
- 3 garlic cloves; minced
- 2 tbsp. rosemary; chopped.
- 1 tsp. fennel; ground
- Salt and black pepper to the taste

Directions:

1. In your food processor mix garlic with fennel seeds, fennel, rosemary, red pepper, some black pepper and the olive oil and blend until you obtain a paste.

2. Spread 2 tbsp. garlic paste on pork loin, rub well, season with salt and pepper, introduce

in your preheated air fryer and cook at 350 °F, for 30 minutes.

3. Reduce heat to 300 °F and cook for 15 minutes more. Slice pork, divide among plates and serve.

Nutrition Values: Calories: 300; Fat: 14; Fiber: 9; Carbs: 26; Protein: 22

Beef Brisket and Onion Sauce Recipe

Preparation Time: 2 hours 10 Minutes

Servings: 6

Ingredients:

- 1 lb. yellow onion; chopped
- 4 lbs. beef brisket
- 8 earl grey tea bags
- 1/2 lb. celery; chopped.
- 1 lb. carrot; chopped
- Salt and black pepper to the taste
- 4 cups water

For the sauce:

- 16 oz. canned tomatoes; chopped
- 1 lb. sweet onion; chopped
- 1 cup brown sugar
- 8 earl grey tea bags
- 1/2 lb. celery; chopped
- 1 oz. garlic; minced
- 4 oz. vegetable oil

- 1 cup white vinegar

Directions:

1. Put the water in a heat proof dish that fits your air fryer, add 1 lb. onion, 1 lb. carrot, 1/2 lb. celery, salt and pepper; stir and bring to a simmer over medium high heat.

2. Add beef brisket and 8 tea bags; stir, transfer to your air fryer and cook at 300 °F, for 1 hour and 30 minutes.

3. Meanwhile; heat up a pan with the vegetable oil over medium high heat, add 1 lb. onion; stir and sauté for 10 minutes.

4. Add garlic, 1/2 lb. celery, tomatoes, sugar, vinegar, salt, pepper and 8 tea bags; stir, bring to a simmer, cook for 10 minutes and discard tea bags. Transfer beef brisket to a cutting board, slice, divide among plates, drizzle onion sauce all over and serve.

Nutrition Values: Calories: 400; Fat: 12; Fiber: 4; Carbs: 38; Protein: 34

Lamb Shanks and Carrots Recipe

Preparation Time: 55 Minutes

Servings: 4

Ingredients:

- 4 lamb shanks
- 2 tbsp. olive oil
- 1 yellow onion; finely chopped.
- 1 tsp. oregano; dried
- 1 tomato; roughly chopped.
- 2 tbsp. water
- 4 oz. red wine
- 6 carrots; roughly chopped.
- 2 garlic cloves; minced
- 2 tbsp. tomato paste
- Salt and black pepper to the taste

Directions:

1. Season lamb with salt and pepper, rub with oil, put in your air fryer and cook at 360 °F, for 10 minutes.

2. In a pan that fits your air fryer, mix onion with carrots, garlic, tomato paste, tomato, oregano, wine and water and toss.

3. Add lamb, toss, introduce in your air fryer and cook at 370 °F, for 35 minutes. Divide everything on plates and serve.

Nutrition Values: Calories: 432; Fat: 17; Fiber: 8; Carbs: 17; Protein: 43

Marinated Pork Chops and Onions Recipe

Preparation Time: 24 hours 25 Minutes

Servings: 6

Ingredients:

- 2 pork chops
- 1/2 tsp. oregano; dried
- 1/2 tsp. thyme; dried
- 1/4 cup olive oil
- 2 yellow onions; sliced
- 2 garlic cloves; minced
- 2 tsp. mustard
- 1 tsp. sweet paprika
- A pinch of cayenne pepper
- Salt and black pepper to the taste

Directions:

1. In a bowl; mix oil with garlic, mustard, paprika, black pepper, oregano, thyme and cayenne and whisk well.

2. Combine onions with meat and mustard mix, toss to coat, cover and keep in the fridge for 1 day.

3. Transfer meat and onions mix to a pan that fits your air fryer and cook at 360 °F, for 25 minutes.

4. Divide everything on plates and serve.

Nutrition Values: Calories: 384; Fat: 4; Fiber: 4; Carbs: 17; Protein: 25

Beef and Green Onions Marinade Recipe

Preparation Time: 30 Minutes

Servings: 4

Ingredients:

- 1 cup green onion; chopped
- 1 cup soy sauce
- 1/2 cup water
- 1/4 cup sesame seeds
- 5 garlic cloves; minced
- 1 tsp. black pepper
- 1/4 cup brown sugar
- 1 lb. lean beef

Directions:

1. In a bowl; mix onion with soy sauce, water, sugar, garlic, sesame seeds and pepper, whisk, add meat, toss and leave aside for 10 minutes.

2. Drain beef, transfer to your preheated air fryer and cook at 390 °F, for 20 minutes.

Slice, divide among plates and serve with a side salad.

Nutrition Values: Calories: 329; Fat: 8; Fiber: 12; Carbs: 26; Protein: 22

Rib Eye Steak Recipe

Preparation Time: 30 Minutes

Servings: 4

Ingredients:

- 2 lbs. rib eye steak
- Salt and black pepper to the taste
- 1 tbsp. olive oil

For the rub:

- 3 tbsp. sweet paprika
- 1 tbsp. brown sugar
- 1 tbsp. cumin; ground
- 2 tbsp. onion powder
- 2 tbsp. oregano; dried
- 2 tbsp. garlic powder
- 1 tbsp. rosemary; dried

Directions:

1. In a bowl; mix paprika with onion and garlic powder, sugar, oregano, rosemary, salt, pepper and cumin; stir and rub steak with this mix.

2. Season steak with salt and pepper, rub again with the oil, put in your air fryer and cook at 400 °F, for 20 minutes; flipping them halfway. Transfer steak to a cutting board, slice and serve with a side salad.

Nutrition Values: Calories: 320; Fat: 8; Fiber: 7; Carbs: 22; Protein: 21

Beef Strips with Snow Peas and Mushrooms Recipe

Preparation Time: 32 Minutes

Servings: 2

Ingredients:

- 7 oz. snow peas

- 2 tbsp. soy sauce

- 2 beef steaks; cut into strips

- 8 oz. white mushrooms; halved

- 1 yellow onion; cut into rings

- 1 tsp. olive oil

- Salt and black pepper to the taste

Directions:

1. In a bowl; mix olive oil with soy sauce, whisk, add beef strips and toss.

2. In another bowl, mix snow peas, onion and mushrooms with salt, pepper and the oil, toss well, put in a pan that fits your air fryer and cook at 350 °F, for 16 minutes.

3. Add beef strips to the pan as well and cook at 400 °F, for 6 minutes more.

4. Divide everything on plates and serve.

Nutrition Values: Calories: 235; Fat: 8; Fiber: 2; Carbs: 22; Protein: 24

Oriental Fried Lamb Recipe

Preparation Time: 52 Minutes

Servings: 8

Ingredients:

- 2 ½ lbs. lamb shoulder; chopped.
- 3 tbsp. honey
- 3 oz. almonds; peeled and chopped.
- 9 oz. plumps; pitted
- 8 oz. veggie stock
- 2 yellow onions; chopped
- 2 garlic cloves; minced
- 1 tsp. cumin powder
- 1 tsp. turmeric powder
- 1 tsp. ginger powder
- 1 tsp. cinnamon powder
- Salt and black pepper to the tastes
- 3 tbsp. olive oil

Directions:

1. In a bowl; mix cinnamon powder with ginger, cumin, turmeric, garlic, olive oil and

lamb, toss to coat, place in your preheated air fryer and cook at 350 °F, for 8 minutes.

2. Transfer meat to a dish that fits your air fryer, add onions, stock, honey and plums; stir, introduce in your air fryer and cook at 350 °F, for 35 minutes. Divide everything on plates and serve with almond sprinkled on top.

Nutrition Values: Calories: 432; Fat: 23; Fiber: 6; Carbs: 30; Protein: 20

Greek Beef Meatballs Salad Recipe

Preparation Time: 20 Minutes

Servings: 6

Ingredients:

- 17 oz. beef; ground
- 1 yellow onion; grated
- 5 bread slices; cubed
- 2 garlic cloves; minced
- 1/4 cup mint; chopped.
- 2 ½ tsp. oregano; dried
- 1/4 cup milk
- 1 egg; whisked
- 1/4 cup parsley; chopped.
- Salt and black pepper to the taste
- 1 tbsp. olive oil
- 7 oz. cherry tomatoes; halved
- 1 cup baby spinach
- 1 ½ tbsp. lemon juice
- 7 oz. Greek yogurt
- Cooking spray

Directions:

1. Put torn bread In a bowl; add milk, soak for a few minutes; squeeze and transfer to another bowl.

2. Add beef, egg, salt, pepper, oregano, mint, parsley, garlic and onion; stir and shape medium meatballs out of this mix.

3. Spray them with cooking spray, place them in your air fryer and cook at 370 °F, for 10 minutes.

4. In a salad bowl, mix spinach with cucumber and tomato. Add meatballs, the oil, some salt, pepper, lemon juice and yogurt, toss and serve.

Nutrition Values: Calories: 200; Fat: 4; Fiber: 8; Carbs: 13; Protein: 27

Beef and Cabbage Mix Recipe

Preparation Time: 50 Minutes

Servings: 6

Ingredients:

- 2 ½ lbs. beef brisket
- 1 cup beef stock
- 3 garlic cloves; chopped
- 4 carrots; chopped
- 2 bay leaves
- 1 cabbage head; cut into medium wedges
- 3 turnips; cut into quarters
- Salt and black pepper to the taste

Directions:

1. Put beef brisket and stock in a large pan that fits your air fryer, season beef with salt and pepper, add garlic and bay leaves, carrots, cabbage, potatoes and turnips, toss, introduce in your air fryer and cook at 360 °F and cook for 40 minutes. Divide among plates and serve.

Nutrition Values: Calories: 353; Fat: 16; Fiber: 7; Carbs: 20; Protein: 24

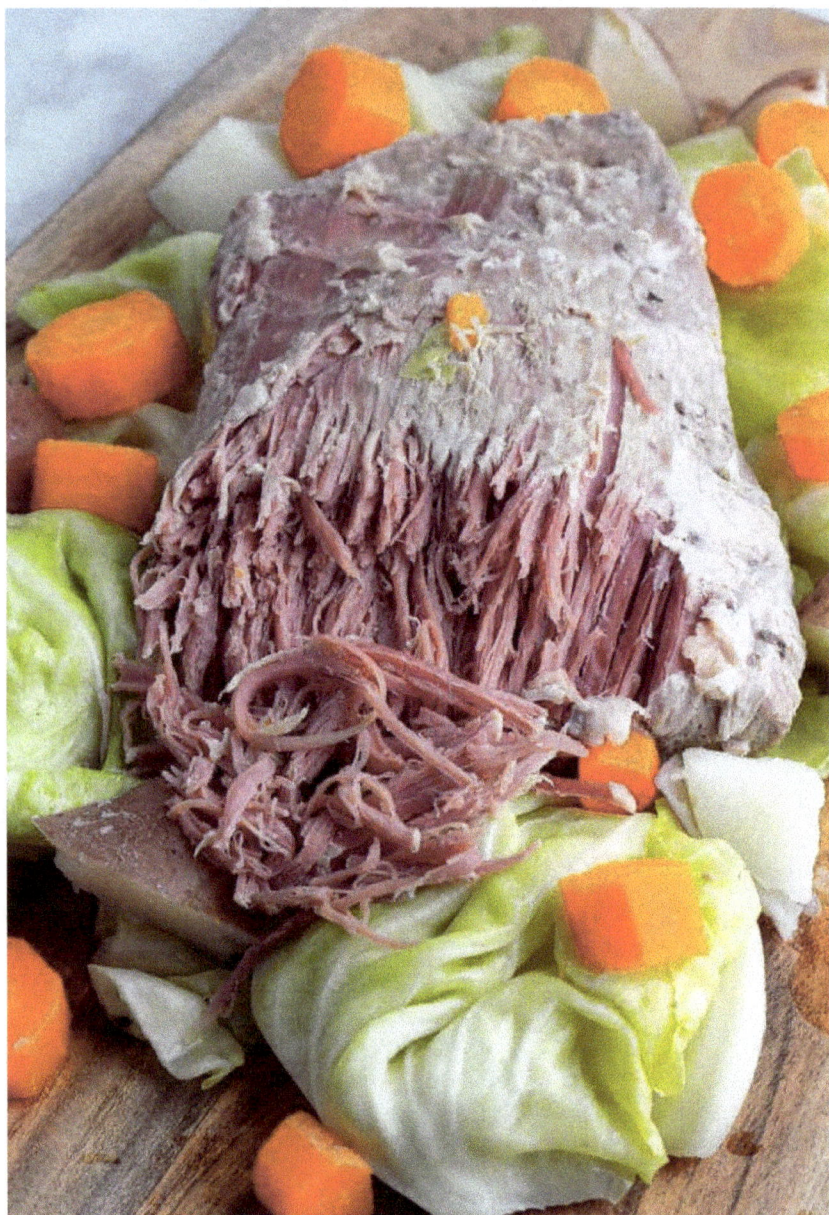